Rapid Weight Loss Hypnosis Mastery

An All Inclusive Walkthrough To Learn How To Dominate Anxiety And Emotional Eating Through Self Hypnosis And Gastric Band To Burn Fat

Self Help for Women Academy

The following Book is reproduced below with the goal of providing information that is as accurate and reliable as possible. Regardless, purchasing this Book can be seen as consent to the fact that both the publisher and the author of this book are in no way experts on the topics discussed within and that any recommendations or suggestions that are made herein are for entertainment purposes only. Professionals should be consulted as needed prior to undertaking any of the action endorsed herein.

This declaration is deemed fair and valid by both the American Bar Association and the Committee of Publishers Association and is legally binding throughout the United States.

Furthermore, the transmission, duplication, or reproduction of any of the following work including specific information will be considered an illegal act irrespective of if it is done electronically or in print. This extends to creating a secondary or tertiary copy of the work or a recorded copy and is only allowed with the express written consent from the Publisher. All additional right reserved.

The information in the following pages is broadly considered a truthful and accurate account of facts and as such, any inattention, use, or misuse of the information in question by the reader will render any resulting actions solely under their purview. There are no scenarios in which the publisher or the original author of this work can be in any fashion deemed liable for any hardship or damages that may befall them after undertaking information described herein.

Additionally, the information in the following pages is intended only for informational purposes and should thus be thought of as universal. As befitting its nature, it is presented without assurance regarding its prolonged validity or interim quality. Trademarks that are mentioned are done without written consent and can in no way be considered an endorsement from the trademark holder.

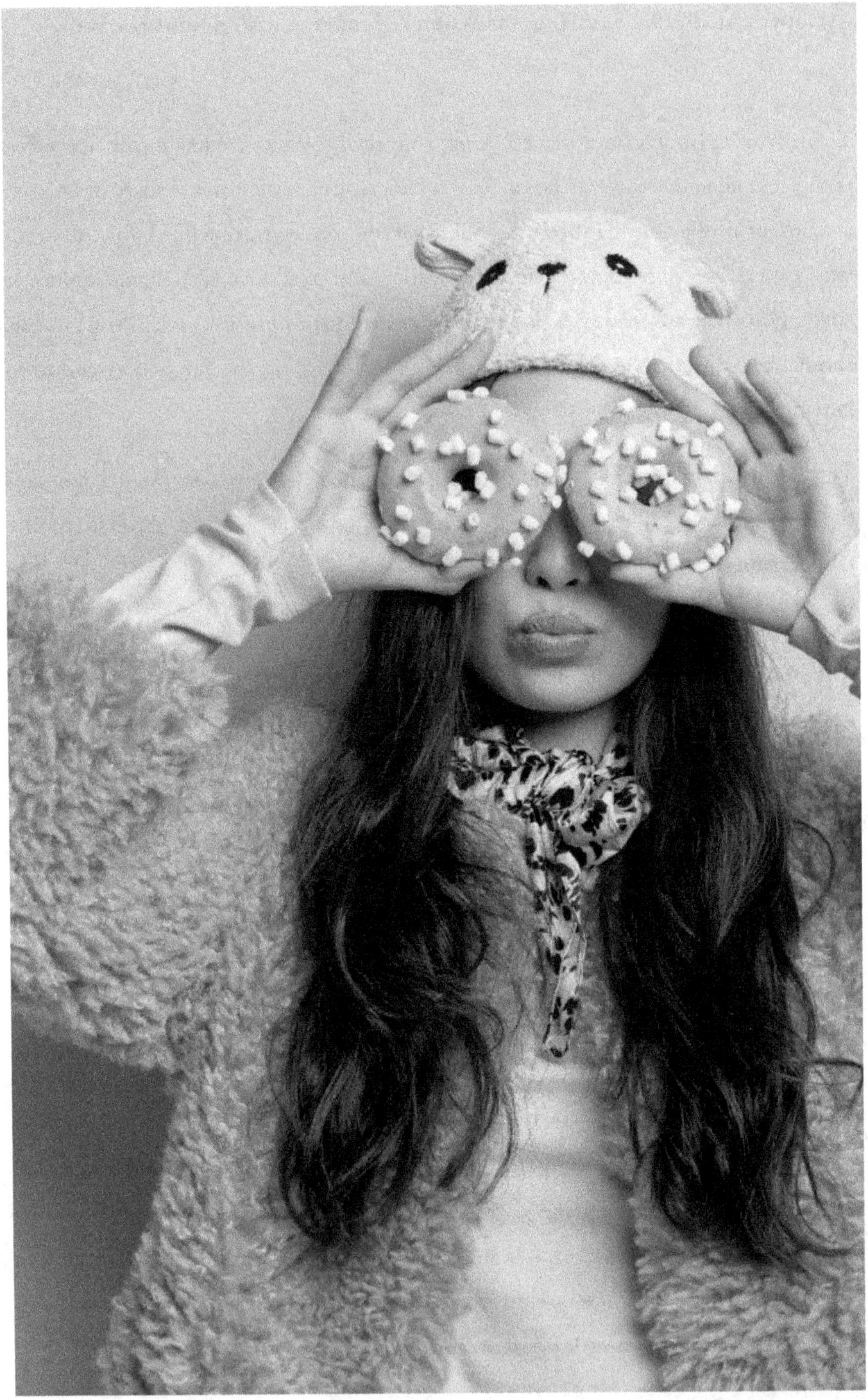

Table of Contents

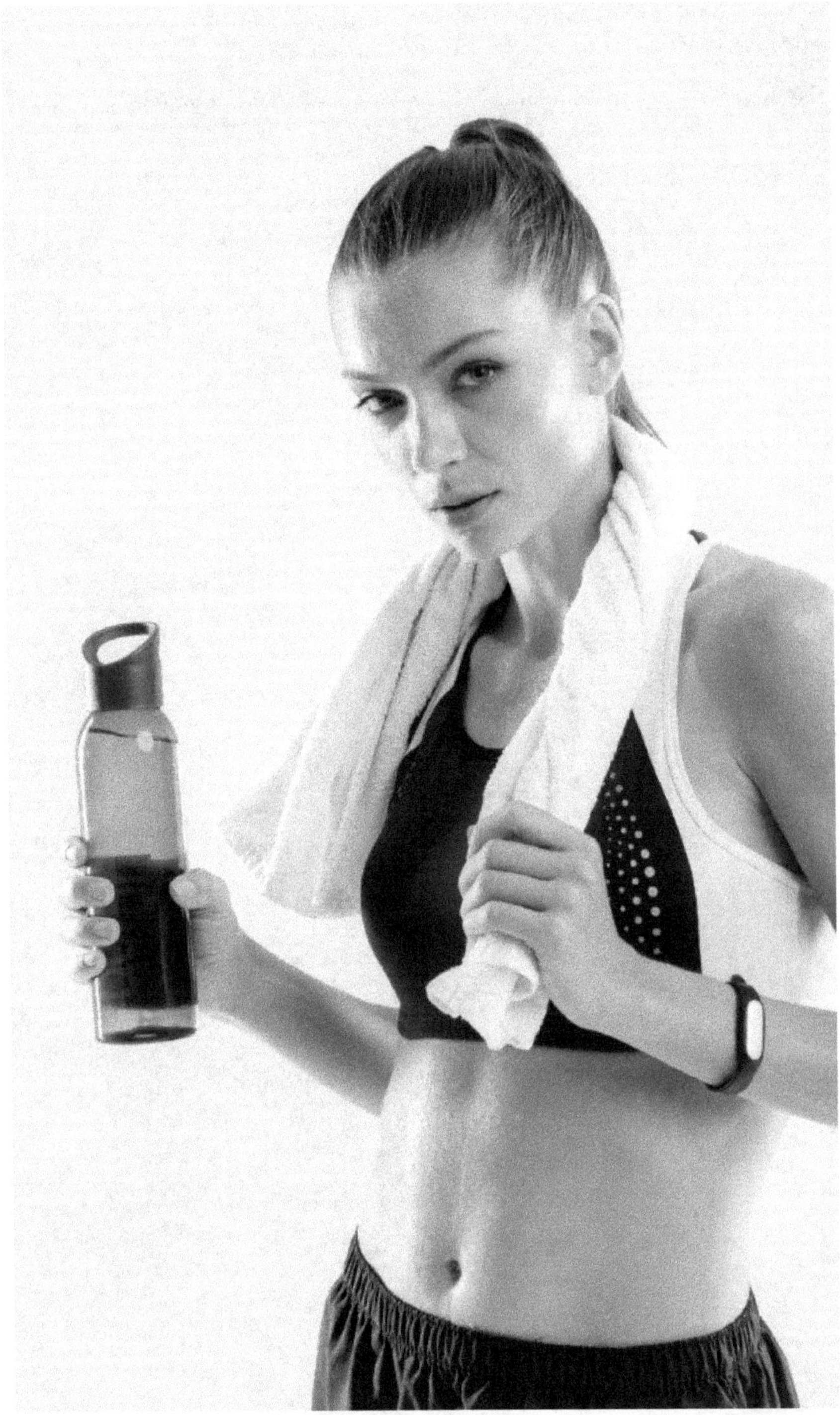

Introduction

This week we spoke with Patricio Lagos, yoga instructor, and director of the trends blog Ansia.cl. He gave us some recommendations to learn to meditate and to use meditation to control anxiety and appetite.

But: What does it take to meditate? Can anyone do it?

PL: All you need is the intention to want to do it, to give yourself the time and space for it. It is not a race or competition. It has to be done willingly, relax, and enjoy.

Yes, anyone can do it, and if you have trouble sitting on the floor for a while, don't worry, you can do it sitting in a chair. The main thing is to be comfortable and relaxed. Although you can meditate lying down, remember that the idea is not to sleep, but be present and attentive.

In your experience, what are the benefits of meditation, and how could it help you maintain a proper weight and avoid overeating?

PL: Meditation is a practice that helps you gain talent to guide the flow of your thoughts. If we talk about taking care of your weight and avoiding overeating, the state of relaxation that meditation produces will lower your anxiety level, leading to bad eating habits. After meditation, the mind is in a state of greater clarity, a state from which we are guided towards naturally beneficial behaviors for our body. When the mind is silenced, the wise voice of the body makes itself heard.

But: If we are trying to eat healthily and face a bar of chocolate or other temptation, how could meditation help us stay in line?

When meditation is done a constant practice, the clarity you get is also based on your decisions and habits of thought and behavior. Don't make chocolate or other temptation your enemy. You have to make peace with how things are because when you stop fighting, it is easier to move in the direction you want to go. Be patient with yourself. You are where you are supposed to be, and you are doing very well.

Give it a try, and you will see how meditation will help you control your weight!

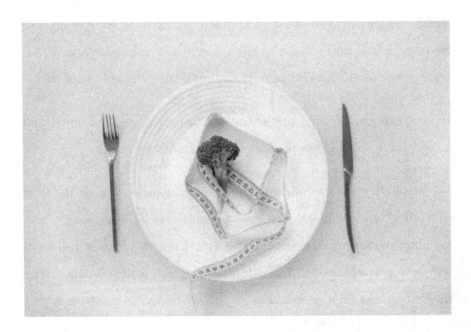

Chapter 1.

Emotional Hunger Tries to Tell You Something, You Must Be Prepared to Interpret It

Being emotionally hungry means being alive, thirsty for desires, projects, and plans. Is there anything more beautiful than feeling alive? Why avoid something that says so much about us?

I hope you join me in exploring what emotional hunger is and all we can learn from it. Ready? Here we go!

What Is Emotional Hunger?

Emotional hunger is a hunger that does not respond to physical hunger but is born in response to psychological needs. When we experience emotional hunger, we tend to crave certain food groups, and we may feel a lack of control when eating them.

Lately, there is a lot of talk about emotional hunger, associating it with stress, worry, or anxiety. Therefore, understanding this hunger as a way to feel relief or a refuge, but the reality is that the equation is not that simple. Emotional hunger responds to many other problems and internal situations whose origin is psychological.

Thus, as an attempt to solve these difficulties (poor emotional management, unresolved conflicts, unsatisfied desires, or needs), food becomes a great ally and companion with a single objective: to help us, and this is done in the short term, so we must learn other different strategies that do not negatively affect.

Therefore, it is essential to understand that healing emotional hunger will allow us to achieve an external change (obesity, overweight). Instead, it will lead us to achieve an internal change and thus transform our relationship with ourselves. So, let's make peace with food, stop viewing it as an enemy, and learn from it.

Learning to Differentiate between Emotional Hunger and Physical Hunger

The main differences between physical hunger and emotional hunger can be summarized in 5:

Causes: physical hunger occurs when our body needs nutrients to continue functioning. Emotional hunger responds to internal conflicts of psychological origin; looking in food for privacy, relief, protection, security, pleasure, disconnection, freedom. Mode of appearance:

physical hunger gradually increases and can wait. Emotional hunger appears suddenly and urgently.

Satiety: physical hunger is much easier to satisfy. After eating, we feel satisfied, and it leaves us satiated for hours. You eat what you need. Emotional hunger is much more challenging to satisfy. We can even feel that I eat what I eat. I will never feel full. You eat more than your body needs.

Choice of foods: when we are experiencing physical hunger, we can decide which foods we choose to nurture our hunger. We are not only satisfied with specific foods and are open to various options. When we experience emotional hunger, we don't have as much power over which foods to choose. They usually satisfy certain foods (sweets, snacks with an intense flavor, fast food, and pasta).

Emotions it generates: after responding to physical hunger, we are left with a feeling of satisfaction, without experiencing unpleasant emotions. After eating emotionally, emotions such as guilt, sadness, frustration, anger appear.

Physical Hunger versus Emotional Hunger

To some extent, we are all emotional eaters (who hasn't found a nook in the stomach for dessert after a sumptuous meal?). However, emotional eating can be a real problem for some people, causing severe weight gain or binge eating cycles.

The problem with emotional eating is that as soon as the pleasure ends, the emotions that trigger it remain, and you often feel worse for having eaten the amount or type of food that you have eaten.

That is why it helps so much to know the differences between physical hunger and purely emotional hunger.

The next time you feel like having a snack, see what kind of hunger is driving your behavior.

Physical hunger:

- Appears gradually and can be delayed

- Can be satisfied with any meal

- You can stop eating when you feel satisfied

- Does not cause feelings of guilt

Emotional hunger:

- You feel an urgent need to eat

- Causes a desire to eat something special (for example, pizza or ice cream)

- You eat more than normal

- Causes a feeling of guilt when finishing eating

- Questions to ask yourself

- You can also ask yourself these questions about your eating behavior:

- Have I been taking more extensive than normal portions?

- Like at unusual hours?

- Do I feel a lack of control over food?

- Am I anxious or nervous about something, like my school, a social situation, or an event where I will be evaluated?

- Has a significant life event happened to me that I am having a hard time coping with?

- Am I overweight, or has my weight gained a lot?

- Are there other people in my family who use food to cope with their emotions?

If you answer yes to any of these questions, it is possible that Eating has become a mechanism for managing emotions rather than a way to fuel your body.

A Craving Is It Emotional Hunger?

A craving is a desire for a specific food. This desire usually appears intensely and urgently, experiencing it with a certain degree of lack of control. Cravings for certain foods are a sign that the body needs stability and calm. The mechanism responsible for this is homeostasis, our body's ability to self-regulate to stay in balance.

Therefore, a craving is a sign of imbalance. There may be different types of imbalances: food, physical, or emotional. When this happens, the body tries to give us signals to seek balance again, but if we ignore it or do not know how to listen to it, cravings appear to regain homeostasis through food.

In short, a craving is a message from our body expressing a need, intensely and urgently. Therefore, rather than looking for culprits (stress, boredom), it would be more interesting to understand what we need.

For example, if you experience stress, your body may need to rest, and the craving for a particular food is an invitation to ask yourself, what do I need now? How could it give me more rest? If you keep working at your usual rhythm, your body will need balance to ask you to eat a particular food to feel better momentarily.

If you experience boredom, instead of food, what other things might your body need? Maybe new experiences, creativity, a desire to connect with yourself. How could you provide what you need?

If you feel sad, it would be interesting to ask yourself what you usually do when you feel that way. What could you do differently instead of eating?

Cravings are messengers that tell us that we are alive and hungry: hunger for ourselves, hunger for love, hunger for movement, hunger for connection, hunger for stillness.

The problem is found when we have to "satisfy" this hunger through food because what came to warn us that we needed something (the craving) can turn into something harmful if we always respond in the same way: food.

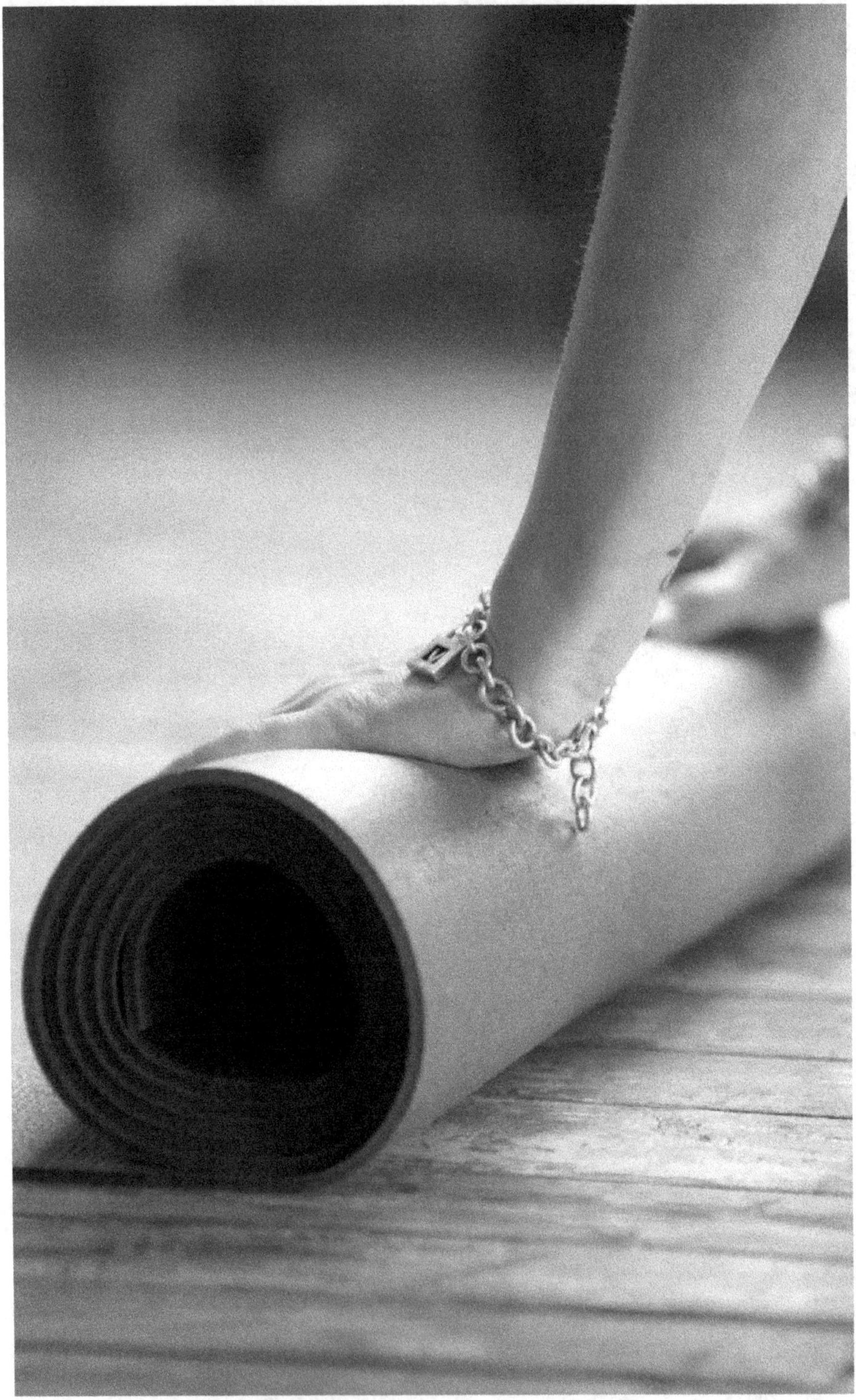

Chapter 2.

Healthy Habits to Lose Weight

B
e it healthy or unhealthy, and a habit is something you do without thinking about it. People who are successful in losing weight make healthy eating a habit.

These healthy eating habits may help in losing weight:

Organize Your Kitchen

- Keep healthy foods in sight. Keep a bowl of fruit on the sideboard and pre-chopped veggies in the refrigerator. When you're hungry, a healthy snack is on hand.

- Reduce temptation. If you know you can't control yourself with cookies, keep these and other diet-spoiling foods out of reach, or even better, out of the house.

- Always eat off the plates. Eating straight out of a container or bag promotes overconsumption of food.

Practice Healthy Eating

- **Have breakfast.** An empty stomach is always an invitation to overeat. Start the day with whole-grain bread or cereal, low-fat milk or yogurt, and a piece of fruit.

- **Plan ahead.** Don't wait until you're hungry to decide what to eat. Plan your meals and go to the market when you feel full. Unhealthy options will be easier to overlook.

- **Turn off the screen.** Eating with your eyes on the television, computer, or any other distracting screen takes your mind off what you're eating. Not only do you lose the taste of food, but you are more prone to overeating.

- **Eat healthy foods first**. Start with some soup or salad, and you will be less hungry when you get to the main course. Just avoid cream-based soups and salad dressings. Eat small snacks often. Instead of 2 or 3 large meals, you can eat smaller meals and healthy snacks to get you through the day.

- **Weigh yourself.** The information on the scale will help you see how your weight goes up or down, depending on your Eating. Keep your home cool. Feeling a little chilly in winter can help you burn more calories than if you keep your house warmer.

Get Help

- Make sure you choose people who understand how important this is, who will support you, and not be judged or trying to tempt you with old eating habits. Submit progress reports. Let your friends know your weight goal and send them weekly updates on how you are doing.

- Use social media. Some mobile apps allow you to record everything you eat and share that with select friends. This can help you keep track and be responsible for what you eat.

Measures That Will Bring You Better Health

On the occasion of World Health Day (April 7), we review the most critical medical recommendations that can help us live in better health and spirits, now and tomorrow.

1. Start running: aerobic activity (such as running) regulates blood pressure, increases lung capacity, reduces stress, and increases bone density. Eat more vegetable protein: these substances provide us with necessary amino acids, lower blood pressure and heart disease, and cancer risk.

2. Sunbathe with care: Vitamin D from the sun can protect us from disease, improve bone health, and prevent depression. Of course, use high factor sunscreen.

3. Drinking coffee: some research indicates that moderate coffee intake (1 cup a day) can combat type 2 diabetes and reduce dementia and heart disease risk.

4. Eat walnuts: a Harvard study found that those who ate walnuts every day were 20% less likely to die from cancer, heart, and respiratory ailments.

5. Using spices: natural seasonings are a healthy alternative to salt and sugar; also, they have anti-inflammatory, digestive, and antioxidant properties (turmeric, cinnamon).

6. Don't smoke: tobacco makes us age faster and damages our genetic code, as well as blood vessels and multi-organ systems.

7. Avoid alcohol: excessive alcohol consumption increases health risks, so it is important to drink in moderation (no more than one glass of red wine a day).

8. Ingesting chilies: hot peppers or chilies can reduce blood pressure levels, thanks to its capsaicin, reducing the risk of strokes.

9. Manage stress: tension increases free radicals, particles that can alter blood pressure and increase the possibility of contracting diseases.

10. Strength exercises: weight-training increases lean muscle mass, improves balance, protects our joints, and strengthens muscles and bones.

11. Eat more vegetables: science has proven that high-fiber diets lower cholesterol levels and lower the risk of heart disease and certain cancers.

12. Be generous: a study conducted with an elderly population showed that those committed to helping and supporting others ended up living longer lives.

13. Eat more fish: eating fatty fish (salmon) at least two times a week can increase your intake of omega-3 fatty acids, which support heart health.

14. Get quality sleep: resting 7-8 hours every night takes care of the immune system and cognitive function. Poor sleep can lead to obesity, heart disease, and depression.

15. Feeling Young: you are as old as you feel, and feeling younger can help you live longer. Experts say that attitude towards aging affects health.

16. Getting up from the chair: any movement you make can prolong your life. Physical inactivity can mean an increased risk of heart disease, cancer, and diabetes.

17. Berry fruits: grapes, tomatoes, or bananas are prominent sources of phytochemicals and antioxidants, helping prevent or delay brain aging.

18. Keep the brain active: stimulating the brain improves cognitive functioning for a longer time (learning new things, participating socially, doing puzzles).

19. Take care of friends: connecting with others helps us enjoy better mental and physical health, even speed recovery, in illness.

20. Copy the Japanese menu: eating many vegetables and fish and stopping before you fill-up could explain why the Japanese have the longest life expectancy in the world.

21. Stretch: stretching and flexibility exercises support joint health, minimize the risk of arthritis, and promote balance, preventing falls.

22. Finding a purpose: when you have something to live for, you can end up staying a little longer. And according to psychologists, creating meaning in life brings happiness and health.

23. Think positive: having a positive vision can help you follow healthy habits (exercise and eat well) and are linked to low inflammation levels.

24. Walking more: according to the European Society of Cardiology, 25 minutes of brisk walking a day can add 3-7 years to life and prevent heart disease, diabetes, and cancer.

25. Being a volunteer: volunteering helps prolong life (if done selflessly) since it can lower blood pressure and reduce stress and depression.

26. Have sex: People who remain sexually active tend to live longer. Since it releases oxytocin (a wellness hormone), it lowers blood pressure and helps you sleep better.

27. Take care of your teeth: healthy teeth can decrease the number of harmful bacteria in the body, promote a more balanced diet, and improve overall health.

28. Ditch soda: There is strong evidence that sugary drinks contribute to diabetes, obesity, metabolic syndrome, and heart disease.

29. Commit: marriage can increase life expectancy, protect us from stress, and improve our risk of developing heart disease, Alzheimer's, or cancer.

30. Be Thankful: focusing on the positives helps us prioritize what's important, reduce stress, and find the motivation to stay active and eat well.

31. Hydrate: water can help the kidneys and liver function optimally, support weight loss, and promote healthier, more youthful skin.

32. Surprise yourself: Astonishment generates positive emotions and can reduce inflammation and lower your risk of heart disease, diabetes, and even Alzheimer's.

33. Taking a Vacation: science says that merely taking a few days' vacation can be a way to live longer because it reduces stress and increases happiness.

34. Eat clean: that is, eat as much natural whole foods and vegetables of all colors as possible, and limit meats, dairy, and sugar.

35. Having a pet: interacting with animals reduces cortisol (stress hormone), increases oxytocin, and lowers blood pressure and cardiovascular risk.

36. Watching cat videos: An Indiana University study found that watching cat videos offered more energy and positivity and offered fewer negative emotions, such as anxiety.

37. Having children: a recent project in Sweden found that men and women lived longer after age 60 if they had children (because of social support).

38. Enjoy grandchildren: in addition to being physically active, grandchildren help you reap social connection benefits.

39. Get regular checkups: regular screening checkups can increase longevity by finding preventable or modifiable diseases in childhood.

40. Connect with nature: people living in areas with more vegetation and green areas have a 12% lower mortality rate.

41. Maintain a healthy weight: being overweight is associated with some life-shortening health problems, such as heart disease and diabetes.

42. Take calcium: this mineral will help prevent our bones from becoming more brittle over the years. You'll find it in canned fish, milk, and leafy greens.

43. Yes, to Dark Chocolate: it can improve blood lipids by increasing healthy HDL cholesterol levels, protecting the heart, and reducing cancer risk.

44. Meditate: meditation has been found to increase an enzyme that helps protect against cell damage and aging by 30% and improve concentration.

45. Sing: Singing may help immune function and improve heart rate through deep breaths. Also, it has a positive effect on the quality of life. Connect to social media - Staying connected online with social media can improve longevity, as long as you spend time on real support activities.

46. Laughing: deep laughter could be a form of Exercise that lowers arterial stiffness (helping your heart), improve blood sugar, and de-stress.

47. Have plants: filling your house with plants could reduce volatile organic compounds in the environment and lower the risk of neurological disorders and cancer.

48. Time for one: spending time doing activities that you enjoy is a mind-body strategy that helps reduce stress and improve your overall health.

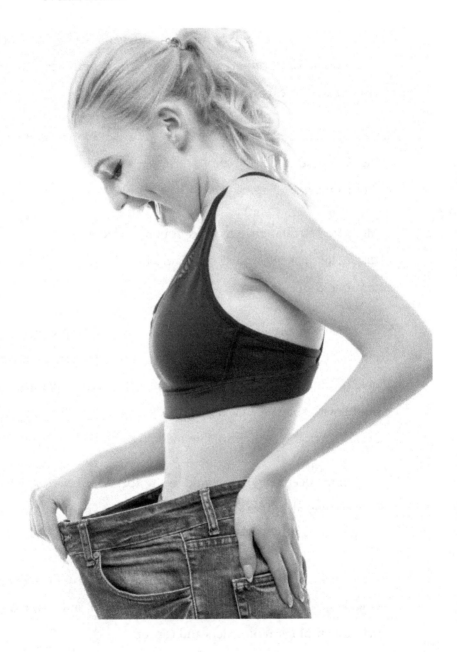

Chapter 3.

The 10 Habits of the Healthy Person

Here is a list of 10 habits that are essential characteristics of the life of a healthy person

1. Sleep

A healthy man respects his rest hours. He does not sleep less than 6 hours or more than 8. Doing the opposite is not healthy. The truth is, when you take care of your sleep timings, you assure your memory of better performance and encourage creativity. Poor sleep care can lead to a myriad of health problems, including your body weight.

2. Avoid Sitting for a Long Time

Dr. David B., who was Steve Jobs' GP, says that sitting for more than five hours straight is the equivalent of smoking a full pack of cigarettes.

3. Watch Your Diet

The healthy man not only takes care of what he eats but how he eats it. This does not imply that from time to time, you cannot eat a treat. The key is balance. It is not about becoming obsessive about the subject and counting calories all day, only to find a middle ground and be more aware of choosing your food.

4. Never Skip Breakfast

And by saying never is never. A healthy man never overlooks breakfast, as it is the most important meal of the day. When you eat breakfast, you start your body's metabolic functions to work correctly during the 16 or more hours that you will be awake. It is not about eating what you find in the pantry. Each meal provides food from the three main groups: fruits, vegetables, cereals, tubers, and animal origin products.

5. Exercise

The correct functioning of a healthy man's body and his quality of life will always go hand in hand with his physical activity. It is nothing new for you, and you already know it, but it is time that this time you put it into practice. It is proven that people who exercise a minimum of 15 minutes a day live an average of three years longer.

6. Drink Lots of Water

A healthy man drinks at least two liters of water every day. Water, in addition to hydrating and detoxifying you, can work as something therapeutic. In Japan, people usually drink a glass of water on an empty stomach to combat severe illnesses and discomforts, such as headache and body pain, arthritis, cardiac arrhythmias, epilepsy, being overweight, bronchitis, asthma, meningitis, kidney, and urinary tract diseases, gastritis, diarrhea, hemorrhoids, diabetes, constipation, cancer, among others.

7. Drink (Alcohol) in Moderation

A healthy man drinks, but he does so in moderation and always remembering that alcohol is to be enjoyed as if it were a rare fad. A good whiskey on the rocks for stress, a mojito, or a beer for the heat, or red wine to accompany the meal never falls terrible. Just try not to make it a habit. Excessive alcohol consumption, in addition to damaging your liver, brings with it heart and cerebrovascular disorders, and generates impotence.

It is clear that it goes without saying, but it doesn't hurt to remind you that a healthy man doesn't smoke either.

8. Keeps Your Mind Sharp

A healthy man laughs a lot, learns more than one language, or listens to music frequently. Just as there are exercises to improve physical performance and keep the body in shape, there are ways to get your mind to stay agile and in good condition. The first are just some examples. Similarly, the consumption of green tea, nuts, and even chocolate is recommended to help your brain's performance improve significantly.

9. It Is Positive

The healthy man is fully aware of the truths behind that old saying: "Healthy mind, healthy body." When worries, stress, or negative emotions are not handled correctly, the body recent everything. It's not about joining the optimists' club or buying the entire library of self-help literature, just about learning how to deal with the daily dilemmas in the best possible way. Another saying that applies a lot to this point is an Arabic proverb that says: "If your problem has a solution, what do you worry about. If you don't have it, what are you worrying about?"

10. Has Frequent Sex

And it does it only because the practice of sex, besides being pleasant, reduces headaches and body pain due to the increase in the level of oxytocin and the release of endorphins. It also reduces the chances of developing prostate cancer, reduces stress, improves your defenses, burns calories, improves mood, and enhances feelings of pleasure and well-being.

Chapter 4.

How to Have a Healthy Relationship with Food

The diet is the fuel necessary for the engine that is our body. Insufficient diet, as well as that which is excessive and unhealthy, can cause severe damage to our body, also unbalancing brain functions

Excesses never get us on the right track, and this idea also extends to food.

We live surrounded by food and exposed to the usual bombardments in our society: advertising, super combos, menus, temptations, hypercaloric foods, eating at the movies, eating in front of the television.

Everything invites us to eat. Simultaneously, we are invaded by the "cannot" by depriving excessive fasting, diets, light proposals, hyper-thin models, books, cosmetics, and thousands of treatments to be thinner every day.

But how are we choosing to achieve a healthy and balanced body and mind? In our conduct is the key.

I Chose to Feel Better

We learn to eat in childhood where, as a normative rule, you can eat everything, with almost no limits between what is healthy and what is not.

However, with development, the formula is reversed at a certain age, and what was allowed before is now forbidden or cannot.

Going to these extremes is not advisable. We well know that diet is the fuel necessary for the engine that is our body. Insufficient nutrition and that which is excessive and unhealthy can cause severe damage to our organism, also unbalancing brain functions.

Therefore, learning to eat wisely, providing the necessary nutrients, and indulging ourselves from time to time should become an immovable rule for every day.

Our environment greatly influences our relationship with nutrition and health. According to Dr. Edith Szlazer, nutritionist and psychologist, one of the keys to understanding the issue is that "dieting is fashionable, and that is copied. Someone starts with a diet, and everyone begins to do it.

The capacity is lost. To realize that the body belongs to one, and it is necessary to take care of it. It is necessary to establish a positive relationship with the body because it is not a receptacle where we put what we want."

The main thing is to learn to choose how to eat and follow some rules for a healthy life: eat very often, learn to eat breakfast, not skip meals, do physical exercise.

Adopting these principles every time we sit at the table is the best way to change our food relationship.

There are times when, when taking care of ourselves with food, control gets out of hand: either we stop eating what our body needs, or we overeat, or sometimes we even engage in very harmful behaviors to achieve unrealistic goals.

Eating disorders are complex diseases that require both a physical and psychological analysis of the person who suffers from them. For the nutritionist Cecilia Ponce, "the success of her recovery is in the holistic treatment, and the family and social support."

Patients with eating disorders are afraid of food; they are afraid of the desire to eat. Within their family, they tend to be perfectionists, to feel underappreciated, abandoned, and alone.

They tend to be part of overprotective and highly structured families and ineffective in solving emerging problems. Furthermore, they are unhappy with their body image and have low self-esteem.

For Dr. Szlazer, one of the factors that influence these symptoms' development is the lack of communication: "The eating disorder is not separated from a culture full of violence, alcohol, drugs a culture where everything is the body, the body is used instead of the word. If we talked more, if we could express our feelings more, we would run that axis, and not everything would be in the body."

In an attempt to maintain weight, unhealthy methods are often used. The most common are excessive fasting, starvation, compulsive eating, and the indiscriminate use of laxatives, weight loss medications, diuretics, or even excessive exercise. An irrational fear of gaining weight and an obsessive desire to lose weight is the first sign of disease.

How to Reverse Them

Given the complexity of the problem, the treatment must be multidisciplinary: medical follow-up for diet, psychological support, physical activity, and family support. It is essential to work on the patient's aspirations, define and visualize who they want to be physically and emotionally, their state of health and the type of life they want to lead.

We can learn to take our needs to eat seriously because physical or emotional needs are worth it, are essential, and make sense. It is the denial of our humanity's needs or aversion to them, leading to self-destruction, dependency, and, ultimately, eating disorder.

These diseases are expressing that something is happening to us and that it comes from before. Therefore, when facing a treatment, the attitudes that add up are from the whole family, from the whole environment. The more love they give you, the more they support you, the more they hold you back, the better you're going to get over it.

Enjoy Every Moment

A healthy life is linked to communication, filling it with unnecessary food and festive projects and experiences. The way we eat is just a reflection of how we live. Who we are is revealed in everything we do? Nobody is perfect, but we can live and enjoy the endeavor: living well, eating with care, with the awareness that what we eat will become part of us, just as our experiences become part of our life.

Ms. Ponce synthesizes her message by stating that we will find the solution "by being generous with our own body and with that of other people, with pleasure and time, tasting each bite and avoiding waste, and enjoying what we do; because every moment can become unique and unrepeatable." Start putting these tips into practice to enjoy a healthier relationship with your body and with yourself.

Food is an integral part of our day-to-day. It provides us with the necessary nutrients that our body needs, but it also fulfills cultural, social, and emotional functions. What does it mean to be a healthy eater? Are you referring to carbohydrates, proteins, and lipids?

Or vitamins, minerals, and fiber? In this note, find out if you have a healthy relationship with food. Eating healthy goes beyond what you serve on your plate. It is about the relationship they have with food.

How you feel and think about your eating habits can be just as important as the food itself. For example, when eating goes hand in hand with stress or guilt, it is not suitable for your body or mind. These are the characteristics of a healthy eater:

He Does Not Live to Eat or Eat to Live

He eats when he has the need when he is hungry without becoming voracious. You will stop eating when you feel satisfied or slightly "full" and will generally avoid eating to the point of feeling full.

You can easily say "no" to repeating dishes because you are no longer hungry, but if you are still hungry or when the food is incredibly delicious, you will happily accept a second course without guilt. He sometimes eats comfort foods, but does not rely on them to ease an emotional burden or get rid of stress.

A Healthy Eater Makes the Right Choices

By being aware of the importance of a correct diet, you will choose foods that make you feel good during and after consuming them. By common sense, your first choice will not be highly processed foods, and as a good habit, you will not eat them frequently. He is used to cooking at home, both elaborate meals and simple things, using fresh vegetables, whole grains, and sometimes for convenience-canned products. When you eat out, you will instinctively choose healthy foods that adhere to your good eating habits by making nutritious and delicious choices. Still, you do not worry about getting out of the ordinary by eating sporadic foods such as pizza, cakes, pasta, for being a special occasion.

Does Not Empower Food to Change He's Usual Diet

You generally eat healthy because you feel good doing it and consider that your diet is an essential pillar of your health. He believes that no food can break his eating habits. For example, it does not enter the vicious circle of "all or nothing" since I already ate a hamburger, I can continue with a large bag of French fries and ice cream for dessert. If I am going to eat junk food, I will well.

He does not make moral judgments about his relationship with food: "Today was a good day because I followed my diet" or "I ruined all my effort to have a soda."

They Are Not Obsessed with Food

They enjoy eating and the process of making a healthy eating plan, but they are not constantly worrying about what they did or did not eat, what they will or will not eat later. He knows that food is an essential and enjoyable part of life, it is not the only thing, and life has many other priorities.

He does not avoid social events because the food they are going to offer is far from his daily diet. Not influenced by fad or miracle diets. The healthy eater eats according to what suits their lifestyle and promotes their health. They do not need to be experimenting with fad diets.

He pays attention to food-related news but is immune to tabloid statements. For example, gluten is the poison of the 21st century, and the population should stop consuming it immediately.

He has the firm belief that no particular form of diet or any dietary supplement is the right one or the solution to all ills. These are some characteristics of having a healthy relationship with food. Remember that no food is wrong. What is terrible is excess. We can enjoy food, even junk on special occasions, just make wise choices and keep in mind that your health comes first.

Seven Tips to Have a Good Relationship with Food

The foods have meaning for each person. They have the power to control not only health but also emotions. Your choice may have a dark side, the constant concern to eat healthily, gain weight, and maintain your consumption.

Eating: A Fight of Pleasure

Most of us have a terrible relationship with food, we make and break diets because we want to control what we eat, but it is a false control, Santillan indicates.

To change the relationship with food favorably, you need to start by identifying what your case is and accepting it; thus, you can take action to feel better about it.

These are some recommendations so you can get it.

1. **Think about the reason.** Maryann Tomovich Jacobsen, a dietitian and author of the book "Fearless Feeding: How to Raise Healthy Eaters from High Chair to High School," explains that people think they overeat are weak.

   But eating habits are not determined by character. Tomovich indicates that it is vital that you think about why you eat as you do. When you understand what is behind the habits, you will stop feeling bad.

2. **Distinguish between emotional and stomach hunger.** Santillan indicates that you must satisfy a real need, not the one generated when you feel tense or under stress. This way, you will eat only when you are hungry and stop eating as soon as you feel satisfied.

3. **Aim and analyze.** Something that can help you identify the real reasons you eat is writing down your thoughts about food, exploring it, and finding out if you see it as "bad" or "good" and why.

   The dietician indicates that research shows that people overestimate calories in foods they perceive as "bad" and underestimate those found in foods they think are "good."

4. **Enjoy your favorite foods.** If you make a list of the five that are your favorites and give yourself "permission" to eat at least one of them every day, you will improve. Tomovich explains that when you know that you can eat any food, your desire to overeat dissipates.

5. **Combine "good" and "bad."** Instead of classifying them into these categories, try to focus and figure out each food plays; Maryann points out that there are right foods for the body's nutrition and others only for enjoyment.

6. **What you eat vs how much you eat.** Many people think that this is what makes the difference in achieving good weight management, but the specialist points out that people have to eat only healthy foods to lose weight, creates a malicious link.

   For this reason, to change your relationship with food favorably, it is better that you learn to eat the right amount of food that your body needs permanently so that you can stay healthy and, at the same time, enjoy eating.

7. **Do it according to your needs.** Tomovich recommends that you eat according to your appetite, take the time to enjoy each bite, that your foods are the ones that satisfy you, and stop when you feel satisfied.

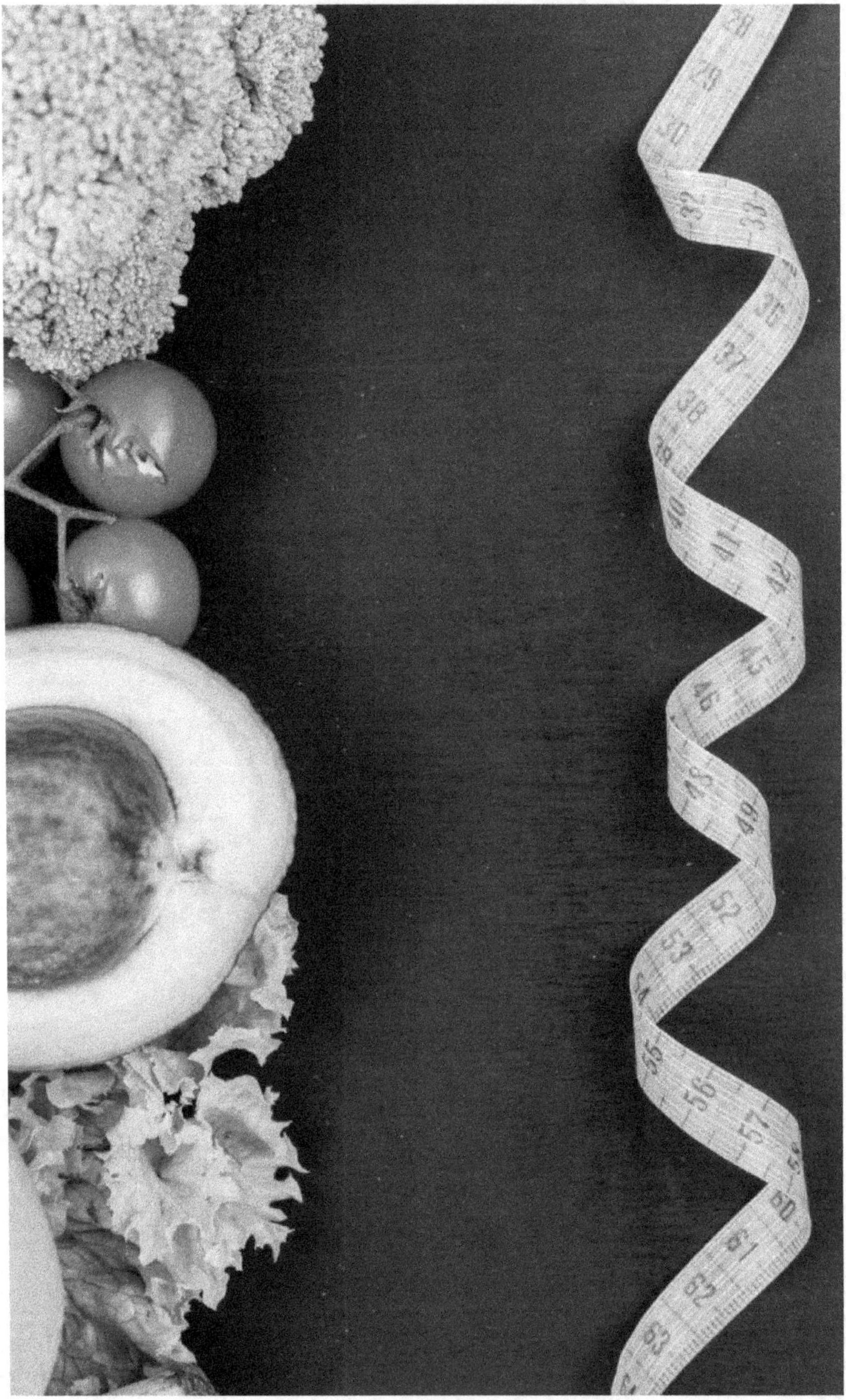

Chapter 5.

The Foundations for a Healthy Relationship with Food Are Laid in Childhood

The relationship we have with food as adults, the more or less healthy habits that we maintain, and the eating mistakes that we make have their origin and their base in childhood.

We talk about emotional hunger, how our childhood experiences influence our relationship with food, and much more.

Many of the eating habits and the relationship we have with food as our childhood learning directly influence adults.

Furthermore, we tend to think that the mood alone influences the relationship with food in adult life.

However, children also experience "emotional hunger." We review, by the hand of Sumati Diez Querol, Nutritional Coach, an expert in emotional hunger management and author of the book "Your relationship with food speaks of you," some of the most frequent questions about eating.

How Does What We Learn in Childhood about Food Mark Us?

We must bear in mind that the relationship with food is created during childhood. "The relationship we have with our mother (the first person who nurtures us), the relationship she has with food, the phrases, and beliefs that are said at home about food, the image we generate about ourselves according to what we say about the way we eat or about our body, etc., creates the relationship that will later be established in our lives, and we will continue as if it were a legacy.

It is easier to create healthy habits in childhood than to change them as adults. Therefore, we can do a lot and take care as much as possible of the relationship that our children have and will have with food," says Diez Querol.

As parents, we are often not aware of the tremendous influence we exert on our children in food and nutrition. Laying a healthy foundation and a healthy relationship also depends on our diet type since we are the mirror in which our children look at themselves.

There are habits that parents have that can negatively influence the eating habits of our children and that we can change. If we share time with them at meals or if they even help us cook, their relationship with food will be healthier: "When they get involved and see it as a creative process, they experience the relationship with food as a game and as something healthy, not as an obligation," says the expert.

Another mistake we make many times is to resort to emotional blackmail: "you will have dessert if you finish what you have on your plate" or "the children of Africa are starving," for example. It is better not to use food as a bargaining chip or as a tool of attack because it can negatively affect it.

What Should We Do to Establish Healthy Food Foundations for Children?

Suppose we want our children to establish a healthy relationship with food and adopt healthy habits.

In that case, it is vital that we set an example and that what we explain and ask them to do, we also comply: "We must try to generate coherence between what we tell them and what we do with food, "says the nutritional coach.

It is also essential the language and the messages they convey, as they have a more significant draft of which we think of the children: "We must pay close attention to the messages that we avoid them sentences of the type:"

In this family, we are trippers, "all women in our family are overweight, "etc.," explains the expert. These messages convey the idea that it is unnecessary to take care of health since it is a characteristic or a family habit.

Keys to Detecting Problems Related to Food in Childhood and Adolescence

It is also essential to pay attention to children's behavior and habits to detect behaviors that may show a health problem or an eating disorder that can increase or worsen over time.

If we act quickly and detect eating problems in childhood, we can correct them sooner. There are some symptoms that, according to Sumati Diez Querol, can give us clues that something is not going well:

- We see them eat more than average, quickly, and without chewing.

- We see them eat less than average and lose weight.

- We must observe the phrases or messages they say about their bodies and their image (self-esteem).

- Observe if they eat to manage emotions (fear, frustration, anxiety, etc.).

"Emotional Hunger" In Children

Mood also influences and affects the relationship that children have with food. It is called "emotional hunger," and it is not just for adults:

"Emotional hunger begins in childhood in many cases. To help them avoid it, we can bear in mind the importance of them being the ones to decide, within a series of healthy foods, what they want to eat and, above all, how much they want to eat.

If we force them to eat more than they want, they separate themselves from the messages of their own body, and the moment of the meal can begin to be related to a screaming moment and stress or trying to be "good kids" if they run out of what they have on their plate.

In this way, they separate themselves from bodily sensations; they do what they are told to do.

One of the keys to ending emotional hunger is to reconnect with those sensations to consciously choose what we want to eat, what the body asks of us, not because of the need to break the rule and what we have been told we have what to do as an act of rebellion "assures the nutritional coach.

What Should We Observe in the Way We Eat to Try to Change What We Are Doing Wrong?

To detect our own "emotional hunger" and try to combat and eliminate negative or wrong eating behaviors is vital that we analyze our habits: "We must observe if we eat when we are physically hungry or if we eat to cover or anesthetize emotions or sensations that make us feel uncomfortable.

To make this difference, we can ask ourselves: would I eat at this moment? An apple (or another fruit, for example)? If the answer is yes, probably what we have is physical hunger, while if the answer is no, indeed, what we have is mental or emotional hunger.

We can also observe if the moment of Eating is an act in itself or if we eat quickly while doing something else (we answer a WhatsApp or work on the computer) and unconsciously.

Eating attentive, even if we eat in 10 minutes, helps us to be more satisfied with food and also, let's make digestion better," advises the expert.

Some of my recommendations are:

Focusing on moderation means having balance. Balance is not about perfection; focus on enjoying everything in moderation rather than forbidding certain foods.

One of the most critical steps is merely making sure you are enjoying your favorite foods in moderation. To put it another way, if you love pasta (and there's no medical reason why you can't eat it), enjoy it in moderation weekly instead of telling yourself you won't eat it and then eat a meal. Emotional eating outburst.

Mindful Eating. Avoid eating alone, in the car, in front of the TV, or while doing something else like reading or writing. To get rid of this, focus on mindful eating. This means sitting down to eat, eating slowly, concentrating on tasting each bite, and not doing other activities like driving, watching TV, reading, or listening to your phone while eating

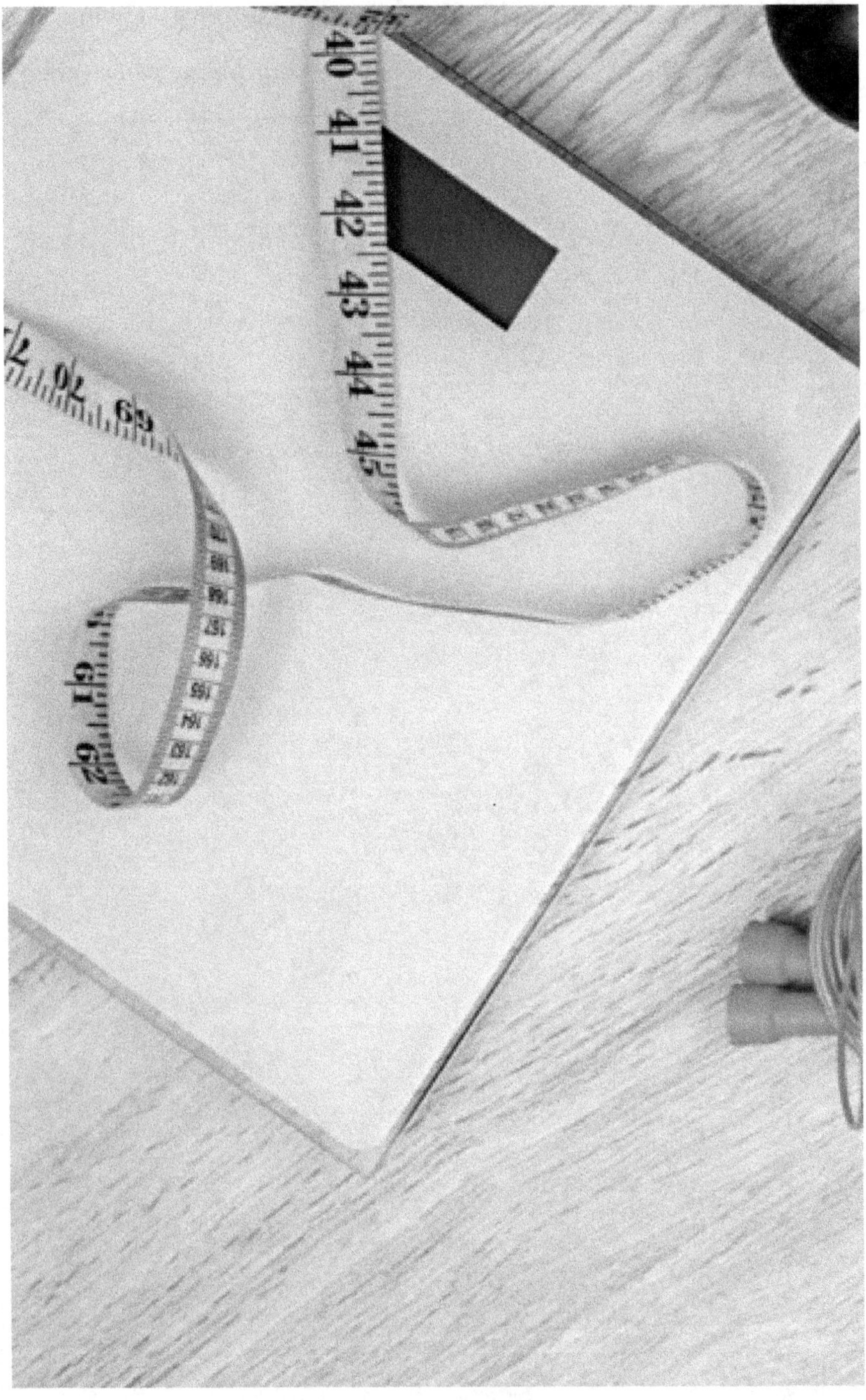

Chapter 6.

Food Addiction, Keys to

Understanding It

Food Addiction

In DSM-5, (5) substance addiction is defined as a maladaptive pattern, leading to clinically significant impairment or distress and is characterized by cognitive, behavioral, and physiological symptoms.

Criteria for diagnosis include tolerance (needing more and more), withdrawal symptoms, considerable time and energy to find, use, and recover from substance abuse, unsuccessful attempts to quit, and continued compulsive use despite the consequences.

Negative and destructive.

What has considered food addiction and the rest of the habits share the pattern of a strong impulse to carry out the problem behavior (cravings or craving), feelings of loss of control over that behavior, and using that behavior to reduce anxiety and avoiding negative emotions?

But other fundamental criteria for substance addiction, such as withdrawal symptoms and physiological tolerance, are not relevant in food.

Scientific Evidence on Food Addiction

First of all, I'll tell you that the idea that a particular food is addictive seems to lack clear scientific evidence to support it. Research advocating the concept of food addiction uses the Yale Food Addiction Scale, which is based on people's felt experience and does not consider food restriction.

We know from neuroscience that when any food is restricted, the reward for that food increases. It is a biological survival mechanism, and people feel "addicted" because they feel out of control about certain foods. However, that is very different from stating that a food substance is physiologically addictive.

Also, the research that sugar stimulates the same brain regions as cocaine or other drugs isn't entirely true.

In studies done in rats, this only occurs under forced deprivation; under these restrictive conditions, the reward response is more significant. Dopaminergic changes that resemble addition only occur with sugar consumption under the intermittent access regimen. Without these conditions, the dopamine response to sugar resembles other natural rewards, such as having sex, taking a walk in the mountains, or doing something we like. When looking at animal research, the only time rodents consume sugar in an "addictive" way is when they have intermittent access to it. When rodents have unlimited access to sugar, they do not exhibit addiction-like behavior.

The critical point to remember is that most foods have an enhanced reward response under restriction and deprivation conditions, both mentally and physically.

There is a large body of neurobiological data suggesting that restriction amplifies the attractiveness and taste of food. Food and drugs indeed share neural pathways, but the brain does not develop a physiological dependence on food substances.

The felt sense of a person out of control or addicted to food is not the same as having scientific evidence that it is occurring on a physiological level. What we do know is that deprivation drives compulsive behavior. Restriction further fuels the feeling of loss of control and a decreased ability to self-regulate. Diet places us in a place of vulnerability to all those foods we are labeling as "bad" or "forbidden."

Why Do We Feel Food Addicted?

As I mentioned, one thing is that addiction to certain foods is not proven as such, or another is that people do not experience the feeling of loss of control and incapacity as something addictive and disabling.

I correctly remember the binge's energy as something that kidnapped me and against which it was impossible to resist.

But it is essential to understand that binges are the result of initially physical and later physical and emotional restriction. When we go on a diet, and our brain detects a condition, survival mechanisms activate the reward system that prompts us to seek urgently food to regain the energy levels to which the body is accustomed. That is, eating too little results in psychological and physiological pressure towards the intake.

Over time and based on repeating restriction actions, it is not only the restriction itself that activates these mechanisms, but only when thinking about it does the brain understand that another limitation is approaching and begins to crave food to prevent the next famine.

So behaviors that look and feel like sugar addiction on the surface are often a function of the diet mindset, which can be just as powerful of a feeling as addiction. Through restriction or "good" or "bad" food labels, food control rules, etc., a real or perceived deprivation is created that can trigger an overriding urge to eat. In other words, the binge occurs in the context of limited access rather than the actual neurochemical effects of sugar.

We generally view eating behavior as controlled by willpower, so when you can't stop eating sugar, it can feel like a personal failure. However, the truth is that it is not a lack of willpower or addiction, but a natural consequence linked to our survival.

The Role of Food in Our Life

On the other hand, indeed, food often takes on a function similar to drugs or alcohol as a form of escape or avoidance.

Thus, we could speak that more addiction to a specific substance, such as sugar, fat, or salt, an obsession or addiction to eating as a way of escape or avoidance.

We often eat to control stress or anxiety. This scenario will indeed sound familiar to you: you have come home after a terrible day at work, maybe you had a conflict with a coworker, or you were stuck on a project.

You start with a pot of ice cream or a bag of chips, and you feel a little better. And before you know it, you've eaten everything.

Many people use food to increase pleasant emotions, such as pleasure, happiness, calm, and uncomfortable feelings, such as anxiety, anger, or sadness. Someone who has experienced trauma in the past may eat comfort foods to cope with feelings of fear, relax, numb, or feel more secure.

Sometimes even obsessive thoughts about food can serve, either consciously or unconsciously, as a distraction from emotions you don't know how to deal with.

Difficulties in our relationships, past or present, can also stimulate an emotional eating pattern. If there has been a shortage of love in your life, you can turn to food to fill the void. Eating can be a source of escape or anesthesia if you are or have been in an abusive or unsatisfying relationship.

It is essential to understand that it is straightforward to use food to cope with feelings and emotions because food is always within our grasp. If we feel distressed, the previous pleasant experience of food leads us to think that we will feel better, eat it, and it works for us: we feel relieved, even if only temporarily.

Therefore, our brain learns that it can get a quick fix and begins a cycle that one can experience as addictive. Foods that are high in sugar, salt, or fat (or all three) trigger a dopamine rush as we see it.

Of course, the problem is that we cannot break the cycle by abstaining from food, as in drugs or alcohol. Since eating is necessary for our survival, the way out of that feeling of eating as an addiction is to become aware of how we use food to regulate our emotions.

The important thing for me is that this perspective creates a space for freedom and no-fault to make more conscious decisions based on a sense of responsibility that the label of "food addict" can nullify.

That is, learning to respond to our emotions instead of reacting to them or placing ourselves in a place of immobility.

Rationally, we know that the void of pain cannot be filled with chocolate cake. We understand that a bag of potato chips will not make us feel genuinely safe or loved. But when we've spent years eating for reasons "other than physiological hunger," it can be easy to lose sight of the proper purpose of food.

It is crucial to differentiate addiction to emotional eating habits. From my personal and professional experience, it is not morally correct to equate both experiences.

What Is the Food Addict Label For?

Finally, I will invite you to reflect on how the label "I am addicted to food" helps you on your way to put peace in your relationship with food.

From a gaze of non-judgment and curiosity, explore whether calling yourself puts you in a place of no responsibility or resignation towards your self-care.

And to finish, don't forget that behind your relationship with food is the relationship with your body. A bad relationship with our body leads us to control or modify it through food or overexertion control. If this resonates with you, I invite you to take a look at my articles on Body Acceptance:

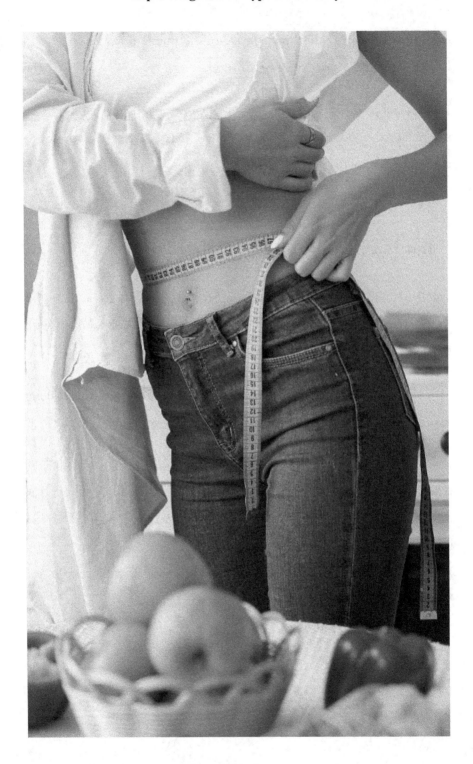

Chapter 7.

Love Your Body Despite

3 Tips to Start Cultivating Body Acceptance This Summer

Just because food and drugs share common neural pathways does not mean that food is addictive. There is no clear evidence to support food addiction.

There is extensive research to support that food restriction leads to overeating and binge eating.

The restriction does not only have to be physical. The emotional or thought regulation can activate compensatory systems. Many people may indeed experience their relationship with food as addictive, but more as a habit, not a real addiction.

Explore how calling yourself a "food addict" helps you take care of yourself. My personal and professional experience is that when we let go of the diet mentality, we give ourselves unconditional permission to eat using mindfulness skills (signs of hunger, fullness, satiety, satisfaction, learning to manage our emotions without food, etc.), and urgency decreases. We can have a good relationship with food.

I Don't Control Food. It Prevents Me

We know anorexia; thanks to it, we also discover bulimia; serious problems cause an eternal obsession with food to revolve around us. But what happens when food controls us?

When we binge-eat and don't purge afterward? Today we will address the lives of all those people who, at certain times in their lives, do not know if they live to eat or eat to live.

Binge-eating disorder identifies those behaviors in which you eat very fast, faster than average, eating food until you feel uncomfortably full, consuming large amounts of food without hunger.

Binge eating affects those who suffer from an imbalance in the brain's reward centers and have low self-control over anxiety. It causes them to become addicted to food, even when they are not hungry.

The consequences are related to their health and emotional well-being: people with this disorder feel guilty and ashamed.

Live to Eat, Eat to Live

Most of us eat to live, and our life does not revolve around food. It is not the case for people with binge eating disorder. For them, their life is at all times, controlled by food. But what is behind all this craving for binge eating?

When we fall into a depression, when we begin to be overwhelmed by emotions, when our self-esteem is on the ground, it is straightforward for us to lose control.

Suddenly, we spin without brake and, without practically realizing it, we begin to reproduce behaviors that destroy us instead of helping us. Losing control is your body's way of telling you that there is something you need to fix. It's getting your attention.

That is why, at times when we are most stressed, with a more excellent range of anxiety, we go to food to try to appease what is corroding us inside. The big problem is that afterward, we don't feel better. Guilt emerges not only because of the number of calories ingested but also because of its quality. Most of the foods will be very unhealthy: chocolate, pizza, hamburgers, and a high caloric load.

"When you develop binge eating disorder, you are not able to fight your cravings for food. It is like an addiction. Cross out the "how." It is an addiction."

Anonymous person interviewed for the Elite Daily.

Binge eating disorder can have different consequences such as obesity, diabetes, chronic fatigue, sleep disorders, and even heart attack risks. Remember that in this disorder, there is no purge. One does not vomit food.

A behavior that is "escape," that in a way "relieves" you, causes your health to be affected. Without a doubt, seeing yourself in these new circumstances can cause a drop in self-esteem, which increases anxiety and the frequency with which bingeing occurs.

We Haven't Completely Lost Control

When you are not able to control food, when the anxiety is so great that you get up, again and again, to calm it with what you find in the fridge, you may think that there is no return, that you will never be able to have control again about those impulses and in general about your life.

As Teo, a man who appeared on the program Samanta Connection, said, "If I don't eat something, I burst. Eating I stop thinking, I avoid all the problems a little, and you say that's it."

Suppose you want to get even closer to this disorder and realize that you have not entirely lost control.

In that case, we leave you this video in which María, our protagonist, explains in detail how to live with a disorder like this.

It is essential to be aware that this perceived lack of control is an illusion. You are perfectly capable of limiting your food intake not to get carried away by such harmful behavior.

The big problem is that you lack the right tools to do it, that you don't know of another way to calm anxiety as fast and easy as eating food. That is why you must go to a specialist.

You eat until you no longer fit in your belly, to the point of wanting to vomit

As Maria told us in the video, food is not the problem. It is what we want to see. We seek to blame food for inquiring about what hurts us and what is causing us to act in this way. It is a way of escaping, of not facing everything that affects us, that we have been dragging along for a long time.

Covering the problem with a new one will not be a solution. It will only make it worse and even cause other types of evils. It is still a way to continue hurting us. In our eagerness to seek relief in food, we self-destruct. The best news is that with a little effort and professional help, you have a solution.

I've Lost Control of Food: These Are the Symptoms

Loss of control over eating is a severe condition that revolves around eating behaviors, which negatively affects health, relationships, or leisure. Thought and emotional patterns are involved and can lead to complete loss of health.

The person begins to focus on weight, food, or body and mobilizes all his energy and all areas of his life to achieve his goals. These same goals are often impossible to achieve and pose a risk to the person in themselves.

Food and its control and its effect on the body begin to create a vicious circle. The person can feel satisfaction at first, but later everything congregates in avoiding discomfort. An effect very similar to that produced by drugs in us.

Disorder or Drug

When we think of a person who has lost control over food, we often imagine someone with an eating disorder, although this is not always the case. Anorexia or bulimia involves more elements besides that loss of control. In some cases, eating has been associated with escaping from discomfort, quickly seeking satisfaction, or only not thinking. It makes us feel right at first, with increasing guilt or sadness appearing. But it implies that we will have a greater tendency to fall back into what we are fleeing from. We eat uncontrollably again, not to feel bad, and we begin to generate a vicious cycle.

The brain processes that accompany addiction processes are the same triggered in those cases where food is a source of avoidance of reality and after the loss of control. A similar mechanism that ends up also bringing very negative consequences for those who suffer it.

So, It Appears

Throughout our lives, we are faced with various situations in which our emotions take on a particular role. There is anxiety, stress, sadness, or guilt. It is a necessary process, but one that sometimes we want to skip. We look for avoidance mechanisms, escapes that we cling to, and that makes us, although only at first, feel good and run away from negative emotions. Food is one of these mechanisms, creating a vicious circle that adds to the initial problems.

The symptoms that make us see that we have been able to lose control of food are the following:

1. Negative Emotions to Food

Whatever it is that made us run away with eating, we have now begun to associate it with being wrong. Everything related to her, we reject, like eating out or cooking.

2. Weight Changes

The physical state is affected, even abruptly, either by gaining or losing weight. The others are also aware of this change.

3. All or Nothing

We can go much of the day without eating, and the moment we taste the food, we cannot stop. We usually associate it with anxiety when there is also a real and physical hunger.

4. Rejection of Our Body

Food and our emotional discomfort impact on our body image, which we will also reject, becoming part of the problem. Food is something we live with daily and is part of our culture.

We know that there is a problem when we reject or deny it and, it is especially notable when guilt or shame also appears before it. Apparent symptoms that tell us that we should seek help.

I'm going to start by asking you a prevailing situation, which I'm sure you will find familiar:

Maybe you want to lose weight, change your habits, or change your lifestyle. You have forbidden yourself to eat sweets. You have committed to eating only real food. You love chocolate, but the one you like the most is not allowed, and you know that it makes you fat. Suddenly, at home or work, you start to feel the anxiety to eat in a moment of boredom or stress, an intense desire to eat sweets, cookies, Chocolate!

Or you've had a long, hard workday, and you tell yourself you deserve an award. You know that what you want is not healthy, that chocolate is full of sugar, and you hear and read everywhere that it is terrible.

You want to stand firm, but you can't take it anymore. You convince yourself that it will only be a small piece. In the end, you eat half a tablet.

After a few seconds, you are filled with guilt and frustration, guilt, and you ask yourself, "why am I not able to do it?"

You get discouraged, although you promise yourself that you will not do it again, although each time you trust less and less.

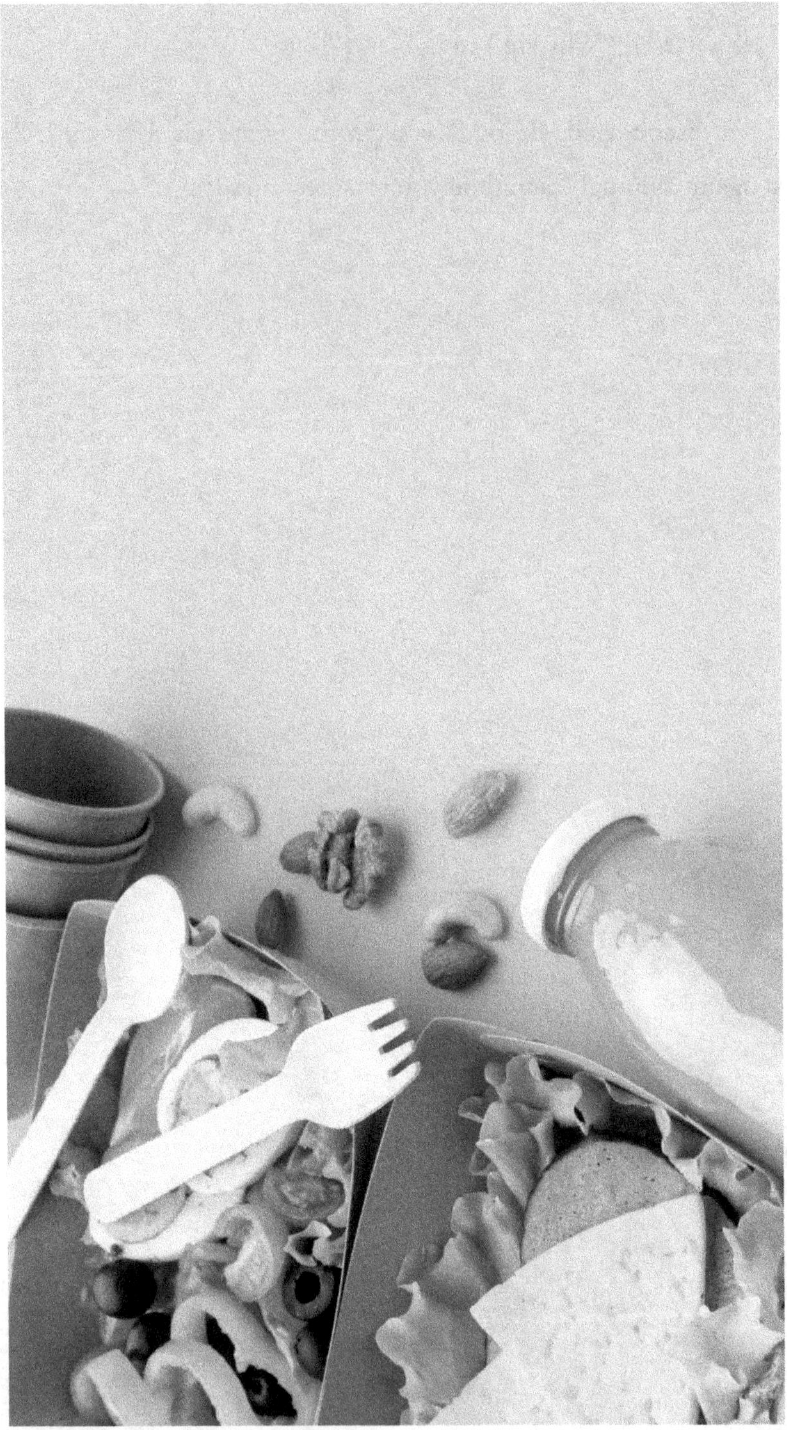

Chapter 8.

The Best Approach

Any activity that requires concentration: sports and leisure activities, painting, singing, sewing, making macramé, or patchwork. Take time for yourself: prepare a warm bath with soothing essential oils such as lavender or make an appointment for a relaxing massage.

A new and Different Approach

Other leisure activities, more trivial, but very therapeutic, reduce stress and anxiety levels: meet a good friend, go dancing, go to the movies, watch a comedy series or a comedy, go with a group of friends to improvisational theater, look for humorous monologues.

We cannot go from disorder to order in one-step. Nor does it feed the deprivation, which leads us to a lack of control. Although I already know that the tendency is to want to go fast, I warn you: not by running a lot, you get there before. Unlike.

With which the strategy is now different: more respectful and sustainable. Step-by-step, we will arrive at the destination. But these changes are very little change! Don't underestimate the power little by little. In the end, we will make a lot!

And since I don't want you to believe me either, I propose that you experiment and be practical: if what you've done has not helped you so far, try something different. So, I encourage you to, instead of removing, add: add nuts to your breakfast, fruit at meals, add fresh vegetables to your meals

"But if I don't take away and add, I'll get fat!"

No! When we add food that meets our body and mind's real needs, little by little, we stop obsessing over food all day. Our cells stop crying out for real nutrients to help keep them alive.

That cry that we translate into anxiety to eat, on many occasions, is nothing more than our cells starving for useful and essential nutrients.

How to put this recommendation into practice?

If you eat a croissant for breakfast, add a fruit and a handful of nuts. If you eat a pasta dish, add a gazpacho or a vegetable salad first with a dessert (no, fruit for dessert is not fattening).

At the same time, if you want to go a step further, try to eat as much as possible as little as possible. It is not the same to eat a cake made by you with natural ingredients than industrial pastries. It is not the same to eat a paella made by you than a pre-cooked one.

- Make sure you consume good quality and quantity fats daily:

One of the most widespread myths that hurt us enormously when it comes to taking care of ourselves "Fat makes you fat." FALSE.

Fat has many functions in our body:

- Repair skin

- Neurons are part of our brain

- Well-being and hormonal balance: It is part of:

    o The hormonal sex

    o The hormones of hunger and satiety: Increase satiety

    o Improves our mood: positive, stable

    o Organs in balance

What Fats to Consume?

All that Mother Nature offers us.

Those that would be convenient to avoid as much as possible or at least for daily consumption would be the ultra-processed and the trans hydrogenated (margarine) and animal products that come from industrial exploitation (that eat feed and that are exploited).

Super Fat

- Virgin olive oil (EVOO) first cold pressing: 5 tablespoons of olive oil.

- Coconut oil: 2 tablespoons daily (you can use it to sweeten the milk).

- Nuts, seeds, and seed creams (tahini).

- Avocado.

- Ecological eggs: 6-7 eggs a week.

- 100% coconut milk.

- Eat complete meals with all foods. Do not remove any type of food.

Fruits and vegetables of all kinds (seasonal and organic), fish (not farmed), whole grains, or pseudo-cereals (brown rice, red, quinoa, buckwheat, amaranth), legumes, seeds (pumpkin, sunflower, flax, sesame), etc.

The lack of some nutrients, such as protein, can cause you to feel hungry shortly after eating.

If you eat a nutrient-poor diet, your cells remain hungry and won't stop asking for food until you give them the nutrients they need.

- Vary your dishes and enjoy healthy food

Food, in addition to nourishing us, has to satisfy us. Lack of pleasure in what you eat can lead to bingeing and pecking. If you take care of yourself or lose weight, you base your daily diet on dishes without flavor or color, and you will not last long. Eating unsatisfactorily is an unsustainable situation for a long time. A week maybe? Or at most a month. And what a month!

The reason is that shortly after eating bland and boring, a series of reactions are unleashed in you: voracious hunger, craving for "forbidden" foods, constant and continuous appetite, desire to peck ultra-processed products that generate explosions of flavor in the mouth.

- Find satisfaction in your life

Our way of living is related to our way of eating. In addition to the lack of pleasure in what we eat, other situations may be related to the lack of joy, satisfaction, and personal fulfillment.

For example, the lack of recognition, feeling valued, or the lack of a life project. We try to make up for these deficiencies with food but only do it momentarily.

When the effect of the flavor wears off, or we digest that dish, we connect again with the internal emptiness.

If we do not have any source of pleasure in our life, if our experience is unsatisfactory, if we have a job, relationships, or studies that we do not fulfill or like, and even if we do not feel satisfied with ourselves, we may end up overeating.

We use food as a desperate attempt to guide our way, fix our shortcomings, and provide us with the pleasure and spark of excitement and satisfaction that we lack in life.

Human beings have basic needs, and among them are satisfaction and pleasure.

Suppose we do not satisfy them in all areas of life. In that case, we will always compensate ourselves in another way, and eating is a resource that we use.

- Record your intakes, emotions, and thoughts

Choose a notebook and always carry it with you. Every morning or night, write down some reflections. You can also do it at other times, such as when you feel anxious to eat or when you feel ravenous hunger. Find your journal and write down how you feel at that moment.

You may feel resistance doing it because, on many occasions, we avoid and reject feeling our emotions out of fear of overflowing, not being able to cope with what we think.

You need to know emotions themselves are harmless. They cannot hurt you. You can feel pain, yes, but a bearable ache.

There is an unbreakable rule of our unconscious that serves to protect us. This is because we will never connect with anything that we cannot bear. So, if you get carried away and connect with an unpleasant emotion, you can be sure that you have the resources to cope with it.

- Invest in yourself: the way out is inward.

I want to tell you something personal: the day came when I realized with my own story that I had only mastered binge eating and purging, controlling behavior based on self-imposed strategies.

But the internal volcano was still active, and the eruption was escaping from other sides: toxic relationships, emotional dependencies, obsessive and self-destructive behaviors, and so on.

It led me to discover that behind the desire to lose weight—whether it was necessary or not—in cases of overweight, obesity, or the inability to follow a dietary pattern, hiding eating disorders, organic imbalances, high levels of stress, discomfort, anxiety and deep emotional background to be resolved.

Moreover, the vast majority of cases were hidden under an apparent lack of will or laziness because not all of them are as obvious or known as anorexia or bulimia.

In the same way, it happened with cases of the other extreme: people who sought perfect health through an obsessive, restrictive, and uncompromising diet.

Although they manifest in different ways, there is a common denominator.

Like the cases of binge eating disorder, food addiction, and so on. Beyond labels and diagnoses, the origins are similar, although each case is a complex, unique and particular universe. And so, should be your approach and your process of recovery, learning, and healing.

Carl Jung already said: "The shoe that suits one person is narrow for another: There is no recipe for life that works well for everyone."

In my research path more than 14 years ago, I discovered the most astonishing revelation: both metabolic disorders, binge-eating, and eating disorders were not problems in themselves, but symptoms that stemmed from internal imbalances or specific needs on a personal level deeper.

They were not external problems but an outward manifestation of internal problems (or imbalances).

Achieving exact and accurate change involves learning, transforming, and integrating. It is not achieved in two days, it requires time, effort, perseverance, love, perseverance, patience, and enthusiasm, but the result will be a great reward.

Changing eating habits and lifestyle is to gain harmony, conquer one's inner balance, which will translate into an outer balance, and restore the emotional bond with food.

To end:

If you want to change your relationship with food, lose, or maintain weight, there must be a change in your consciousness and your personal development.

To do this, you will inevitably have to offer something of yourself. I'm talking about commitment and responsibility, but not from a specific numerical result or physical evidence from day one.

Commitment means doing everything you have to do to achieve it, involving reading, training, meditating, and making the necessary changes in yourself, your environment, and your life.

Taking responsibility and committing ourselves are the indispensable requirements to change our inner world, shape our destiny, regulate our way of eating.

For this, we must take the reins and listen once and for all that learning life has for us, and we will achieve this if we attend to the message and the signals that it indicates to us through the symptoms that we suffer.

Have you ever wondered what you're eating habits hide and why after dieting, you always gain weight or eat poorly again?

Starting an exit inward and attending to the real causes of what happens to us is a long journey back home, not to go to a different place.

It is a journey whose final destination is to recognize you, rediscover yourself, connect with your essence, regain your inner power and say goodbye to that character with whom you have identified and that, deep down, you know that it is not you.

The goal is to connect with the person under those layers of fat, with that lousy mood experienced due to guilt after having binged.

That superb and complete being without that toxic way of eating, without that perpetual obsession, without those self-criticisms that make life better for him and those around him.

"I want to be me again," most of the people I accompany tell me this because, no matter how much we identify with the extra kilos or with a particular way of eating, we deeply know that we are much more than that.

And our true selves are eagerly waiting to be released, recognized, and heard. To achieve all this, you may need to go through a therapeutic process and receive accompaniment, and this is not being weak, on the contrary.

As Brene Brown says, "Recognizing our history and loving ourselves throughout the process is the bravest thing we can ever do."

Eating emotionally, a habit that can be changed with this strategy. How many times have you felt stress, worry, or anxiety? How many of those times did you eat just to feel relief?

On some occasions, more than one of us has taken refuge in food, but when this becomes a habit, it becomes unstoppable, and that is when we begin to depend totally on food to satisfy our emotional needs.

If this happens to you frequently, and you want to change that compulsive habit, pay attention to the following because there is an effective technique to control that impulse over food, and here I explain how.

Have you ever wondered why we have the desire to eat?

It seems like an obvious and natural question, and the best answer is simple: we eat because we are hungry.

What if I told you that it's not just like that?

Eating is a necessary physiological act.

However, the desire to eat can be influenced by many causes, and most of these are not physiological but emotional.

We seek to channel that emotion of anxiety or frustration through the act of eating (thinking that we are hungry). In the simple act of eating and selecting your food, several factors that we all know influence, such as hunger, appetite (craving), income, and the availability of food.

But additionally, your emotions, mood, and feelings of stress or anxiety influence. Food can become a temporary relief to a much deeper problem, feeling, or emotion.

It happens because your brain secretes several powerful substances that produce pleasure (such as dopamine).

This reward is so powerful that your brain will look for any opportunity to motivate you to eat that food that produces pleasure. It is more the simple fact of thinking that food or taste will make the brain have a pleasant sensation. Things get complicated when your brain associates this food or merely the act of eating with a negative emotion or feeling.

For example: "being sad and eating chocolates," "feeling stress and eating cookies," "having anxiety and eating everything and in large quantities." It is for this reason that emotional eating becomes a habit.

Later I will explain how this habit was formed. But first, it is crucial to differentiate emotional hunger from the everyday need that we all feel.

How Can We Differentiate Emotional Hunger from Physiological Hunger?

It causes weight gain and also severe psychological and emotional consequences. Eating something only on a whim is not the same as eating emotionally.

We all have "cravings" for certain foods from time to time, but the behavior is controlled due to a satiety factor. Also, the craving does not involve moods, and it is not a repeated behavior. One way to know if you eat emotionally is by answering the following sentences with a yes or no. It is a professional test and can help you identify the problem.

- I feel out of control in the presence of delicious food

- When I start eating, I can't seem to stop

- It's hard for me to leave food on the plate

- When it comes to food, I have no will power

- I feel so hungry that I can't control myself

- I can't easily satiate myself

- I continually have worried thoughts about eating or not eating

- There are some days when I can't think of anything but food

- Food is always on my mind

This test was taken from a study that developed an index to detect the habit of eating based on reward.

It means the habit of eating based on instant gratification or temporary relief from some emotion.

How Did You Form the Habit of Emotional Eating?

As you read a few paragraphs earlier, your brain associates an emotion or feeling with a mighty reward. In addition to this substance secreted generating pleasure, the feeling of fullness experienced after eating in large quantities can also become a reward that triggers an unstoppable habit known as "binge eating" or "emotional eating." The habit of eating emotionally is triggered as a reflex action to a specific stimulus such as sadness, stress, or anxiety.

First, we have a stimulus that motivates us to eat until we finally find the reward. The only way to change the routine of emotional eating is to recognize that it encourages us to do so and find another pattern that allows us to obtain the same reward.

Why Is It Important to Change That Habit as Soon as Possible?

Physiologically there is an apparent affectation, but on an emotional level, there are serious consequences, and it is precisely at this level that the root of the problem lies.

So, like any other harmful habit (such as smoking), it is imperative to change it since emotional eating inevitably leads us to be overweight or obese and, in other cases, to develop other severe eating disorders, damaging our health.

This habit of emotionally out-of-control eating can compromise the brain's reward pathways, similar to drugs.

If the habit is out of control, you must seek a professional who will evaluate you closely.

How Can I Change the Habit of Emotional Eating?

The objective is to change that routine that hurts you, which generates the same reward but is healthy.

When you feel about eating, distract your mind with another activity. That is, change the routine of this habit to control the urge to eat emotionally.

Here are many strategies to distract your mind and curb the urge to eat emotionally. I want to propose this: the 5-minute process.

This strategy has been used previously by some of the community members regularly (and have had good results).

The 5-Minute Strategy to Stop Eating Emotionally

- What will we need?

- A stopwatch (you can use the mobile one)

- A pen and paper

- Eager to change

Indeed, you already have all these tools so, to explain what it consists of, you must first follow these steps:

- Write in detail the habit you are going to change

The goal in this step is for you to identify and write very specifically about this habit of emotional eating. In this way, you will know very well what is the routine (pattern) you want to change.

Merely writing, "compulsive or emotional eating" is not enough. You have to be more detailed.

For example: "emotionally eating chocolate chip cookies at night when I feel lonely."

Be as specific as you can. The point is that you identify which routine is the one to change.

- Identify precisely what motivates you to start eating

This step can take several days; you have to identify what exactly motivates you to start eating. What is the object, feeling, emotion, person, or situation? That encourages you to start eating. Each person is different, and the remainder is unique. Eye! It is not the same as trying to explain why you eat emotionally. The objective is to identify the key that motivates you to start that routine.

To make it easier, when you feel the sudden urge to start eating, you have to ask yourself these five questions for several days to do an analysis.

- Place: Where am I?

- Time: What time is it?

- Emotional state: How do I feel?

- Feeling of hunger: Am I hungry or not?

- People around: Who is around you?

- Immediate Prior Action: What were you doing at the time?

Always carry a note on your mobile or a notebook, as you must write it down when you have the urge.

At the end of this analysis, you will be able to identify a pattern. Maybe it's your emotional state, or perhaps it's at a particular time, or even a person that makes you nervous.

The goal is to find what motivates you to start eating, that is, your reminder.

It also gives you a little time to your advantage to slow the momentum, which brings us to the next step.

Conclusion

After having deepened the historical course and the vicissitudes that hypnosis has encountered over time, one might wonder, among others, what this discipline currently represents for the medical and scientific community in general, what they are and whether there are models and techniques of intervention and what are the areas of intervention of the same.

Weight-loss hypnosis can help you lose a few extra pounds when it's part of a weight loss plan that includes diet, exercise, and counseling. However, it's hard to put it definitively because there's not enough concrete scientific evidence about hypnosis to lose weight only. Hypnosis is a state of absorption and internal concentration, such as being in a trance. Hypnosis is usually performed with the help of a hypnotherapist through oral repetition and mental imaging.

When you're under hypnosis, your attention is highly focused, and you respond better to suggestions, including behavioral changes that can help you lose weight.

Some studies have evaluated the use of hypnosis for weight loss. Most studies showed only mild weight loss, with an average loss of approximately 6 pounds (2.7 kilograms) over 18 months. However, the quality of some of these studies has been questioned, making it challenging to determine hypnosis's actual effectiveness for weight loss. However, a recent study, which showed only modest weight loss results, found that patients receiving hypnosis had lower rates of inflammation, better satiety, and better quality of life. These could be mechanisms by which hypnosis could influence weight. Additional studies are needed to understand the potential role of hypnosis in weight management fully.

In general, the best way to lose weight is with diet and exercise. If you've tried dieting and exercise but still have difficulty reaching your weight loss goal, talk to your health care provider about other lifestyle choices or lifestyle changes you can make. Relying only on weight loss hypnosis probably won't lead to significant weight loss, but using it as a complement to a general lifestyle approach may help explore some people.

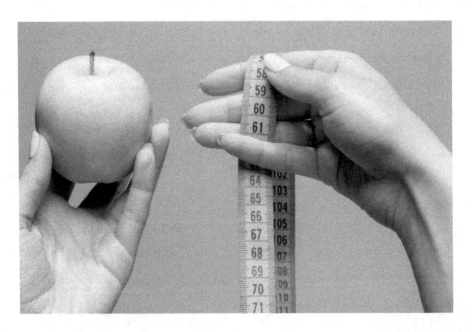

CPSIA information can be obtained
at www.ICGtesting.com
Printed in the USA
BVHW091354210621
610121BV00017B/542